Natural Nubian

P.O. Box 354212

Palm Coast, FL. 32135

Nubia's Organic Hair Guide

ISBN-13:978-1539955221

ISBN-10:1539955222

Rewrite 11/6/2016

Because of the dynamics of the Internet, any web addresses or links contained

in this book may have changed since publication and may no longer be valid.

The viewers expressed in this work are solely those of the author.

Table of Contents

The Organic Guide to Hair Care

The organic path to natural hair care is essential to the hair care. The natural hair community is interested in homemade mixtures because it is more beneficial for all hair and overall health. Finding a resourceful guide to help them understand more about different oils is important, therefore this guide help you gain some simply knowledge about the oils and understand the importance of product awareness. The organic approach to hair care is no longer a trend. It is essential to our wellbeing!

My first book *Nubia's Organic Hair Care Guide* provides my journey and searched for knowledge about hair care. Everyone's transition is different and I share secrets behind my transition from the Cream Crack.

This mini guide provides oil care and nutritional requirements for healthy hair. By bridging the gaps between medical science and the hair care community, we can leverage your path to longevity.

This book is a simple resource tool to help improve daily hair care.

Charles Nessler, a German hair stylist was known for his invention of the perm and curling tools. It was said that he used cow urine and water as the first process that changed the hair ph to an alkaline. Perms are caustic, they burn, and destroy the hair's natural acidic ph. Creating volume and lots of curls was his goal. Changing the hair ph and altering its natural state is known as creating a perm. Nestle's method of the perm combined with a Grateau method – a method involves heating the hair at 212 degrees.

Nestle used his wife for experimentally perming and curling the hair. Unfortunately, Nestle's-wife lost her hair through burns. This process of perming the hair became England's reference in the hair care industry. Nestle's wife patience and his determination set the stage for the hair care industry across the continental United States.

Another inventor, Garrett Augustus Morgan, a child of a former slave from Kentucky, accidently discovered the first hair relaxer for African Americans. This handsome, charming gentleman worked in a factory where discovered that the chemicals he used to repair a sewing machine somehow relaxed curly hair. He tested his chemical on an Airedale dog — a dog that has a curly-matted coated hair. He found the chemicals used for repairing the sewing machine straightened the dog's hair. Tormenting the poor dog by reversing the dog's matted hair to straight fur. Today Mr. Morgan would be charged with animal cruelty!

In 1913, G.A. Morgan went on to expand his business to straighten or relax hair. His company was known as G.A. Morgan Hair Refining Company.

He produced other prominent inventions well-known to the black community, like tools to promote that sleek, European look.

In 1890 Madame CJ Walker worked in a laundry house. She suffered from alopecia, which is a scalp disorder leading to hair loss. Madame Walker manufactured the scalp conditioning and healing formula. Her growth serum and hair care products contain Sulfur.

Although she was the daughter of a slave from the south, she became the first millionaire for her hair care solution. Madame Walker married at an early age, but her age and the past had no bearing to her influence as an entrepreneur and inventor. Madame CJ Walker was also known as Sarah Breedlove. She was the originator of the hair care and beauty industry for African Americans. Her product campaign read, "have a reason to envy another girl, her lovely hair, and her charming complexion." I find this advertisement concerning because it became a misrepresentation of our true heritage. Madame CJ Walker's hair care products promoted growth because they contained potent antibacterial agent known as Sulfur.

In 1910, she traveled to Kentucky in search of the factory needed to expand her business. It's interesting that she went to the hometown of the inventor of the relaxer- Garrett Morgan. She relocated to Kentucky to expand her business.

This prominent business woman influenced Garrett Morgan. Morgan launched his company three years after Madame CJ Walker moved her business to Kentucky. The first perm was an extremely harsh alkaline product that caused the destruction of the bonds of the hair and caused the hair's normal pH of 3-5 to change the pH to 10-13. Garrett Morgan needed a way to reduce the damage from the relaxer. Madame CJ Walker had a solution! In 1905, Madame Walker invented a conditioning treatment for straightening hair.

In 1945 Marjorie Joyner, a graduate of Bethune-Cookman College, joined forces with Dr. Mary McLeod Bethune to improve the hair care industry. Marjorie invented the permanent wave machine, while employed by Madame CJ Walker. This machine straightened black hair and added extended curls to the hair. Marjorie Joyner never received the patent for the permanent wave machine; it remains the property of Madam CJ Walker's Company.

Dr. Mary Mcleod Bethune and Marjorie Joyner partnered to begin the United Beauty School, which focused on the development and the quality of hair care industry.

Perms for some people produced curl, while relaxers straighten hair for others. Either, way the two inventions change the structure of our hair and create a unique look.

Nestle and Garrett both influenced chemical burns and destruction to the hair. Today, we must re-evaluate and understand our hair care needs. Self-acceptance is imperative! Reviewing history is vital because it helps us understanding how to improve on our hair care regimen.

.

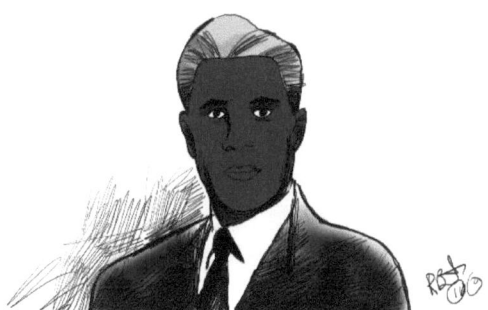

Inventor Garrett Augustus Morgan, a child of a former slave from Kentucky, accidently discovered the first hair relaxer for African Americans.

Our hair is unique! Some people have long hair, some have short hair, some hair is curly, and some hair is straight hair, but one common factor we share is that all hair is made up of protein and has a low ph. or acidic in nature.

Hair grows in 3 phases; it is said our hair grows about 1- 1/2 inch of hair each month.

Anagen Phase

This is the new growth phase in this phase. 3-5 years- people can stay in this phase and normally people with long hair are in this phase. The question is how do we remain in this phase or stimulate hair to stay in this phase?

Catagen Phase

This is known as a resting cycle. And it is the shortest period, lasting only about a couple of weeks

Telogen Phase.

This phase is the cycle most of us remain in, in a resting phase of hair growth and notice no hair growth and lots of shedding. Unfortunate for people who try to grow their hair because the hair pushes the old hair out and causes shedding. It is known to only last 3-6 months.

And the Telogen phase which most of us are stuck at this stage because we do not notice our hair growing at an accelerated rate. No matter what phase you most hair grows about one half inch per month.

My curly sisters may be questioning what phase they are in! But the truth is if we took care of our hair and maintain a balance our hair should grow. Stress, alopecia, and medication are factors we cannot seem to change, but adding a little protein, drinking plenty of water, proper hair care, exercising, and taking vitamins can help.

Source Milady's Standard Cosmetology (c) 2004

Interesting alopecia is a derivative of the Greek word fox- a fox sheds its coat two times a year.

* Everyone was not designed to have shoulder length hair! *But using some simple organic tips from this guide will improve your health. Stop spending all your money on products that do not work for you! Now, this does not mean all manufactured products are dangerous, but your chemical addiction and unrealistic expectations may be the real problem for your hair.

Shampoo or not

Washing your hair is critical, but the question is what do I use?

From *Nubia's Guide to Going Natu*ral, I share that a lady admitted to not shampooing in the traditional methods. She used vinegar, baking soda, black soap, and other mixtures to clean her scalp.

Now dreaded hair is often hair we refer to as if we should or should not because their hair seems to grow at an accelerated rate with or without shampooing. Dread hair does not shed, not like loose hair! And most dread haircare is simple but consistent. They don't apply a lot of junk! The shampooing techniques keep their hair clean. The fact remains that your scalp should be stimulated, clean, and never neglected.

Shampoo may strip your hair of oil, cause more dryness, and increase breakage. Finding an organic shampoo that works well is a challenge, and there is no simple answer because what works for one does not necessarily work for the other. Read the labels, understand possible drug and hair care interactions, and understand the side effects. Yes, these are words from a medical clinician!

Scalp stimulation increases blood flow, and shampooing is necessary for that reason. Adding essential oils, like peppermint and rosemary stimulates your circulation and enhances the blood flow, so adding it to your shampoo will help improve growth for most people. Shampooing is a process when a person is cleaning their hair. Water is the most important part of the cleaning process. Water is a compound containing hydrogen and oxygen atoms, the oxygen compound and molecules are required for all living cells. If you avoid shampooing or even wetting your hair you may become more susceptible to poor scalp conditions and a head full of dead hair?

One important thing you need to know about the shampooing process is the goal is to clean the scalp, remove excess oil, dirt, remove yeast, bacteria, and fungus. During the process never shampoo or tangle your hair using circular techniques, this may create more tangling to the ends of your hair. Hot water is a not good for your scalp, and it is recommended that you use lukewarm to wash your hair then rinse with cold water. Cold water seals the cuticles and reduces frizz of curly hair. Avoid being a lather Queen from your favorite commercial. Focus on hydration and stimulation.

For ultimate cleaning, detoxing, conditioning, and to improve your shine try Aztec clay or Bentonite Clay. Bentonite is an excellent way to remove toxins and clarify your scalp. Try mixing bentonite clay for cleaning your hair, adding your favorite oil, water, vinegar, or Aloe Vera, fragrance, baking soda, and conditioner with Bentonite clay to cleanse your hair. You will have elongated curls and softened curls after the use of Bentonite clay mixture. When using Bentonite clay mask avoid the use of metals because metal fragments will reduce the potential effects of the bentonite. Products build up and become less of a challenge when you use bentonite clay to clean your hair. Bentonite masks used overnight have been known to improve your health and/ or reduce dandruff, so I highly suggest you try it or even add a teaspoon each time to your favorite conditioners for doing the cowash.

Cowash is condition washing your hair without the use of shampoo. It is a great method for skipping the traditional oil stripping effect of shampoo, and it can help improve the texture and shine of your hair.

Prepoo is preparing your hair for shampooing. To prepoo saturate your hair with your favorite oil the night before, covering it with a bag. The next day shampoo the hair. Then the no-poo, I totally do not agree with applying alcohol, corn starch, cocoa powder, baby powder, hair spray and other applications to avoid the cleansing process with water. Some people with extremely oily hair skip the traditional shampooing and apply oil strippers, use the no poo method. Skipping the washing in some cases, if you are sick, are in the hospital, are dealing with infection, or surgery. People who have oily hair can try lemon and other citrus blends to reduce the oil buildup.

Cocainamide DEA has been proven to cause Cancer. Cocainamide is a derivative of coconut that is used commonly to make foam and for shampoos and body wash.

The FDA has just produced the effects of the shampoos containing Cocainamide. You must learn to read the labels before attempting to use these products.

Some products that contain more Cocainamide are:

Mitchell, Palmolive, Sof n Pretty, crème of nature, Do Gro, Design Essentials, American Crew...

For more information, please go to Center for environmental health or ceh.org.

Other product stabilizers and form boosters increase the risk of cancer including Cocamide,

MEA, and DEA- Cetyl Phosphate, DEA oleth-3 Phosphate, Lauramide DEA, Linoleamide MEA,

Myristamide DEA, Oleamide DEA, Stearamide MEA, TEA- Lauryl Sulfate, and Triethanolamine.

FDA recently posted this information, and you need to be aware of cancer-causing agents. A natural way of life includes avoidance of preservatives and other hazardous factory-made chemicals. Read your labels or try mixing your own products.

1. Sodium Laurent Sulfate -This chemical is known to be cancer-causing or carcinogen, and you will find this is a variety of shampoos. The FDA has recently posted multiple warnings about this foam aiding chemical in the shampoos because of its significant risk and potential problems for your skin and eyes.

2. Methylchloroisothiazolinone is one of the worst preservatives. This additive makes the products last longer on the shelf and reverses the real effects of the products. You will not only find it in hair care products, but in cosmetics also. It has been banned and restricted in some areas across the United States.
3. Ammonium Chloride is not digestible and may cause eye irritations. It may cause severe damage to your respiratory tract if inhaled. Propylene Glycol is a great moisturizer and used for your GI tract, but it is harmful to your respiratory system and has been linked to disorders and auto-immune problems in children.
4. Strong Fragrance or Perfumes- are not good in any way. They do cause severe allergic reaction and add no benefits to your hair.

http://site.thegreenlifeonline.org/2012/04/30/finding-a-safe-shampoo- and-what- ingredients-to-avoid/

Understanding porosity is necessary for all hair care and how our hair accepts the water for hydration and oil for moistening, and protein. Dandruff may easily be confused with porosity problems, especially if your hair can not absorb products because the cuticles are sealed too tight.

To determine if you have high porous verses low porous hair, I recommend you get a clear glass of water and put some of your clean hair that shed into a glass of water. If there is any product on the hair, this simple test will not be accurate so make sure the hair is clean and free of any product.

Allow the hair to sit into the water for at least 40-60 seconds and if the hair goes to the bottom of the water that means your hair is high porous. Hair that floats is low porous hair, which means the hair may appear shiny and healthy, but product and water don't penetrate easily, and this hair is more susceptible to breakage and destruction.

Low porous hair is simply hair that has a problem with hydration and moisture balance. This type of hair lacks elasticity and is easy to break. Avoid deep conditioners and protein because it will improve the manageability of your hair. Low porous hair simply does not require more protein because it is full of tightly coiled protein strands. The cuticles are tightly compressed and resist any water or oil going into the cuticle.

The best solution for low porous hair is to spray with water and then oil it. A daily spray of water reduces the tension to the hair and improves your ability to hold moisturizing products to seal the cuticles.

Think about oil in water. If water is present oil is more prominent and it seals the hair shaft. Coconut, Glycerin, Aloe Vera, and steam conditioning help. Find other humectants added to products that help your hair maintain both the moisture and hydration.

Hair porosity should be (medium) to high porous hair) Commonly, the hair may feel soft, you will notice less breakage, and when you apply your favorite hair care product and oils, your hair will not be dry and absorb the products.

 High or low porous hair can alter into a medium porous hair, which is the goal. I've noticed in the past that some people chemically process or dye their hair to open the cuticles enough to allow the moisture and protein to adhere to the hair for easier styling. Finding a more organic solution to porosity problems is a better option. Because dyeing and applying a chemical can cause permanent imbalances to the hair follicle and therefore yield more hair loss.

The best solution again is trying water and then oil if your hair is not high porous. If the hair is high porous, the hydration and moisture is not a real problem. The high porous hair on the contrast has the cuticles more open. This hair is dull looking and needs more oil and protein to keep the cuticles from falling out. Styling is less complicated, and the hair is more flexible. Moisturizing Shampoo, Aloe Vera mixtures, and hydrolyzed protein are the best solution for this low porous hair. Again, protein, conditioners are the best option for the high porous hair.

Simple Steps for Hair Growth:

1. Avoid the heat!
2. Deep condition!
3. Trim your hair regularly.
4. Avoid harsh shampoos.
5. Use liquid leave-in conditioners.
6. Protect and seal your ends.
7. Drink plenty of water.
8. Find a hobby
9. Exercise!
10. Use vitamins enriched with Biotin.
11. Be patient!
12. Protect your hair at night and wear your satin bonnet.

Research and <u>read all product</u> labels before applying these dangerous chemicals to your hair. Chemicals we use daily for hair care may cause diseases like Alzheimer's, prostate cancer, uterine cancer, fibroids, and more.

Any uses of preservatives or genetically engineered products place you at greater risk for the disease. Parabens, Cocamide, and Sulfates are the most common preservatives; they create a great lather and make our shampoos condusive for purchase at our local retail store. Look for words like:

- Methylparaben,
- Ethylparaben,
- Propylparaben,
- Butylparaben they are all different forms of Parabens.

Parabens are found in most cosmetic products. Any small amounts of any man- made chemicals are never a great source for beauty enhancements. Cocamide DEA is a viscosity booster, foam booster, and stabilizer, skin protectant. Sulfates cross the blood brain barrier and any residues left on your hair. The health risk is a primary concern with any use of these chemicals.

Sulfates are the cleansing additives that cause hair to be stripped of its natural oil. Any reduction in the oil creates some effects on curl pattern and causes breakage. Even the smallest fragment of exposure to Sulfates may not create as high of a risk for disease and cancer as most. It is highly recommended that you avoid the chemicals. Maintaining your natural hair appearance, luster and softness can be managed without manufactured chemicals.

Other products we must be aware of are Formaldehyde. It can cause cancer. Formaldehyde is commonly found in chemical strengtheners, silkeners, and smoothners. Formaldehyde 's hard to avoid because it is often found not just in beauty products, but it may be found in food sources also. The risk is greater for exposure because it breaks down and is evolved into the air. High levels of exposure will increase the risk for cancer. Any form of formaldehyde in your silkeners and smoothers with heat added enhances the risk of exposure to the toxins left in the air and may increase your risk for cancers.

Recent studies have linked Leukemia and Lymphoma to the use of permanent dark hair color dyes. Warning hair colors or dyes may increase a delayed anaphylaxis. An allergic reaction can occur after chronic use of hair coloring, and this may become detrimental especially after several years of usage.

There has been more data shared in a new study to show that people who work around the dyes and dye their hair more are often at greater risk for bladder cancer as well as other types of cancer. At any cost, the risk of cancer is greater with the use of any of the manmade chemicals, and I encourage you to understand the risk and take proper precautions. Consider Henna for a safe hair coloring option. The plant-based protein will enhance hair growth if it is used correctly.

Phthalates are used to make shampoos and other beauty products pliable. Phthalates increase the risk to male infants, can cause low hormone levels, and genital concerns.

Parabens are used to preserve your moisturizers, and it has been linked to cancer and breast tumors. Vitamin C and Vitamin E are great safe options to reserve hair products. This information was provided by WebMD 5/9/2014 reviewed by Debra Jaliman-www.webmd.com/beauty/makeup/ss/slideshow-truth-about-beauty-product-dangers

Alcohol, fragrance, petroleum, and wax increase the risk for damage to your hair follicle. They interfere with your goals for long healthy hair. There are much more products that may not be good for your hair, so read your label, research, and avoid all additives to prevent risk of cancer.

Jojoba Oil is a humectant that works great to reduce damage ends and moisturize your hair.

Grapeseed Oil moisturizes and conditions your hair.

Aztec Clay- **like Bentonite clay or Red Clay** (detoxify your scalp), contain electrolytes such as calcium.

Black Soap is one of the best natural cleansers,

Shea Butter adds moisture and softens the hair,

Rosemary and Mint (stimulates hair growth by improving circulation and they are great to reduce hair dandruff.)

Vinegar is ideal for lowering the hair ph. It is a great antimicrobial, and antifungal agent

Baking Soda is a great neutralizing cleanser, reduces odor, reduces oil, and other product buildup.

The easiest way to detoxify or cleanse you scalp is to mix Bentonite clay with ACV- Apple cider vinegar, and your oil of choice. I mix it with my favorite conditioner. Clay mixed with your condition helps soften and elongate curls. Bentonite clay is only sold at select locations.

Black Soap for Hair

Black soap is great for eczema, skin conditions, scalp condition, psoriasis, rash, insect bites, wound care, and scalp sensitivities. African black soap is great for antibacterial, antioxidant, antifungal, antiseptic, and anti-inflammatory and antiviral properties. It is organic and contains minerals and vitamins. Enriched with Vitamin E, black soap is healthy for hair and skin.

It is recommended you purchase black soap from Africa, directly. Be aware that all black colored soaps are not necessarily authentic. The soap is mostly brown, uneven in texture, soft, flexible, and uneven tone. It appears messy in your bathroom, so after usage, it is suggested you dry it and store it in a cool dark area. If kept properly stored it can last longer.

Black soap is, by far, one of my favorite clarifiers because it has an amazing lather and smells good. Soak your black soap in purified or distilled water and add coconut oil or Shea butter. Be careful not to store your hand -made shampoo mixture of black soap because it can create a mold or possibly build up a fungus in your scalp.

Preservative-free products mix with water have no shelf life, so there is no guarantee that the mixture will last. Mix enough to use for one-time use only.

Wash your hair with the mixed black soap, oil, and water. Then it is recommended to use an acid rinse after using black soap to help seal and close the cuticles. The most frequent used acid rinse would be vinegar to help lower your ph. Some woman testifies that the black soap left their hair feeling deprived of oils and adding coconut, or Shea butter helps reduce the oil stripping from your hair.

Good nutrition, drinking plenty of water, and adding vitamins contribute to strengthening your hair. Your hair growth is not determined by what you eat, but how your body responds to what you eat. Hair is living cells and requires essential vitamins. Adding supplements are a great benefit if you are a vegetarian, on medications, pregnant, or have poor nutritional status. All vitamins work together to balance our nutritional needs and requirements for healing and repair of our hair.

Vitamin A is commonly found in your orange-colored fruits or vegetables like carrots, squash, sweet potato, apricots, and cantaloupe.

- It is great for promoting hair growth and thickening of the hair.
- It increases the WBC, the bones, vision, and help with endothelial cell growth. This vitamin taking alone will not significantly change your hair growth.
- Combined with Biotin, Vitamin E, Omega enriched Vitamins, and proteins- Vitamin A will improve your hair growth.

This information was provided by www.hsph.harvard.edu Dr. DJ Frank Michael, H Serum retinal levels and the risk of fracture. N Eng. J Med. 2003 348: 287-294

Vitamin C acts as a hair growth aid and booster. It is commonly found in oranges.

- Collagen with Vitamin C helps build elasticity in your hair. Footnote 1

I've heard people taking baby shampoo and crushing Vitamin C, which is Ascorbic acid to change hair color and to lift the cuticles. Any acid like lemon would potentially modify the hair color by two shades.

Vitamin C taken alone typically has little to no effect on the stimulation of hair growth, but it is necessary for collagen synthesis and certain connective tissue diseases like Scurvy and Rheumatoid Arthritis.

- All vitamins play a significant role in nutritional needs and requirements.

Vitamin D is crucial in the different phases of hair growth. Vitamin D is a precursor to all growth cycles, and the liver converts it into Calcitriol. Our body needs Calcium and Calcitriol for the development of good strong, healthy hair. Vitamin D, Calcium, and Calcitriol control and regulates the follicles by stimulating the cells. Without Vitamin D, the cells die, and hair follicle will become weaken and shed. Foods rich in Vitamin D include Salmon, eggs, tuna, mushrooms, milk, and other dairy products. Vitamin D supplements are imperative if you suffer from chronic fatigue, weakness, and have aching muscles.

Vitamin D is supplied through sun rays, although too much sun and exposure to Vitamin D can be toxic.

Vitamin B complex helps with autoimmune conditions and diseases that affect your bones, joints, or other parts of your body. B Vitamins supports our body's ability to deal with stress. B complex vitamins aid in hair growth. Remember trauma and stress to your scalp require Vitamin B to help it recover appropriately. Vitamin B is produced in many forms:

- Vitamin B12,
- Pantothenate,
- Vitamin B 5,
- Riboflavin,
- Vitamin B 6
- And more

Protein or amino acids are the building block that help with hormone regulations, blood cell growth, enzymes, and new tissue. Protein replaces the old dead cells and produces new healthy cells. Eating of meats and beans increases protein imbalances.

Without protein, our hair will not grow, although the hair itself is a protein, and there are multiple types of proteins. Lysine, Cysteine, and Methionine are all-important factors that increase proteins for hair growth. Lysine helps our body transport the protein and other valuable chemicals to the hair follicle, which aid in the growth. Foods rich in Lysine are chicken, beef, and beans. All forms of Lysine like L-Cysteine and L-Methionine contain Sulfur. Yes, chicken and beans are essential for our hair.

Sulfur is antimicrobial agents that speeds up tissue repair and helps our bodies make Keratin. Keratin is simply a protein. Eating protein helps hair recover and repair from any damage.

Also, try some beans and meats to help build up protein. Our bodies require at least 70 grams of protein or more depending on

weight for cell growth. Check vitamin labels to ensure that enough protein for daily consumption. Footnote 15

Vitamin K helps our body clot and improves hair growth. Green leafy vegetables help with the clotting factors and help stimulate healthy hair. Biotin, Vitamin D, and collagen promote hair growth. Collagen is an amino acid or protein.

Selecting the correct oil is imperative to hair growth. All oils are not created equally. Educate yourself about the different oils. Some oils are great for shine, some are better for growth, some oils help speed up the healing process, and some oils contribute to improving the scalp appearance. I studied the difference between the unsaturated versus the saturated, and monounsaturated oils to determine the truth depth of what that means in the natural hair world. Do you understand some oils are strictly for coating the hair and shine, but they will never enter the shaft or cuticle and may not be your best hair growth option?

- Sunflower oil,
- Canola,
- Mineral oils are not great oils to help improve hair growth.

Sunflower, Canola, and Mineral oil only sit on the outer core or shaft and never enter the cortex of your hair.

Try to avoid mixing too many oils together when you first transition to natural to avoid potential allergies to your hair and scalp. Also, be aware of the difference between essential oils, and carrier oils.

Hair food is extremely important for hair, and we must make sure to add a little shine to help reduce breakage. So many oils can be used to help the hair grow, and you must find the perfect oil blend that works best for you. Digestible Oil work best, and they enhance the sleek and shiny appearance to your hair. Before investing in any oils, research the oils to determine what works best to meet your needs.

Rosemary oil is amazing for growth. It has a pleasant aroma and is known to delay the graying process of your hair. Rosemary leaves an invigorating feeling to the scalp with a light tingling sensation. It stimulates the scalp and follicle which aids in growth and relieves itching. Foot note 27

- Has a pleasant, but herbal, sweet smell and can easily be used as a scalp aroma therapy.

Scrubbing and massaging the scalp with the essential oil will help improve scalp stimulation and improve growth. You may even notice thickening of the hair and increase follicles with the use of rosemary.   Rosemary is inexpensive, and one drop goes a long way. I highly recommend you apply it directly to the scalp without mixing any other oils.   Make sure you select high-grade essential Rosemary oil.

Using rosemary or peppermint essential oils with the inversion method and scalp massages will improve your growth oils.

Other effects of Rosemary are:

- Improve your digestive system
- Rich in antioxidants
- Anti-inflammatory, antimicrobial, antiviral, etc.…
- Improves your neurological effects
- Prevent brain aging
- Reduce cancer
- Protection against macular degeneration
- Watch your migraine headaches improve
- Warning vomiting, spasm, pulmonary edema are potential risk for Rosemary

- Avoid use of rosemary if you are under the care of a physician or if you are taking anticoagulation medication, Ace, lithium, or diuretics.

This information was supplied by the Medical News Today- Sept 5, 21014 by Joseph Nordqvist

Peppermint oil adds great moisturizer that acts as an astringent commonly used to help the scalp by producing a tingling sensation. This oil helps heal scalp problems like dandruff. Peppermint oil helps correct pH imbalances. Ph imbalances can cause a real problem with dryness. Footnote 5

- Peppermint oil smells great, and it has so many benefits I could publish another book to explain the benefits.

You can apply peppermint oil with a carrier oil like coconut oil and other carrier oils and still great full benefits. You can apply it directly to the scalp, drink it, inhale it and still get all the advantages of it.

Peppermint improves:

- Digestive system
- Sleep
- Stress, hair growth
- Thyroid condition
- Reduce migraines
- Increase blood flow and circulation
- It has also been said to help improve the purification process of the water we drink.

Jojoba oil is one of my favorite oils. Jojoba oil helps speeds up the healing process. This oil is like the natural oil our scalp. Jojoba does not spoil and mixes well with other oils. It is great for hydration of the scalp. Jojoba oil adds elasticity, shine, and softens the hair. Jojoba oil seals protects and helps prevent further damage from heat application. Although jojoba oil is not cheap, a little bit goes a long way, and this oil is like your natural oil. This oil is great for reducing frizz and unmanageable hair. Jojoba is a great hair growth stimulant. Try mixing it with avocado oil, coconut oil, and your favorite conditioner for a deep conditioning treatment or pre-poo. This improves and softens your hair. The use of this oil combination regularly for six months or greater you should notice a healthy head of hair.

It is a monounsaturated fatty acid which contains:

- Vitamin A
- Vitamin B1
- Vitamin B2
- Vitamin B6
- Vitamin E

Jojoba oil is very high in fats and strengthens your hair follicles.

- This oil is not cheap, but it mixes well with other oils, and it is a great carrier oil.

Wheat germ oil is not commonly used oil for natural hair, but we must understand it has a great benefit for natural hair. Wheat germ is enriched with Vitamin E. It is great for the prevention of cancer.

I suppose you may be asking the question why antioxidant or anticancer causing properties in any hair care product is relevant. Hair, like the skin, is considered a living microorganism that grows rapidly. Any living cell growth is important; some cells are cancerous, and our body can develop tumors or cancer anywhere. The antioxidant properties in wheat germ are great in the reduction of the spread of unhealthy rapid growing cells to our head, brain, or scalp. Wheat germ also contains Vitamin B, which is perfect for the stress response and for poorly nourished cells that are rapidly growing in the scalp. It helps with new cell development and helps promote rapid hair growth. Foot note 28

- To be very honest, I cannot tell you that this oil is an excellent topical source, but ingested it can give you more benefits to reducing disease.

Aloe Vera is an emergency 911 treatment. Aloe Vera is a repairing oil. It is great for the repair of split ends. Apply oils to the end shaft, and you will notice a major difference in growth and in the appearance of your ends. It can spoil if discolorations are noticed.

I do not recommend purchasing Aloe in bulk. Aloe requires refrigeration. You can freeze it, but be warned that freezing the gel metamorphoses the gel form into a liquid. The gel works better for styling than the liquid. Aloe is great for repair of any damage and helps reduce hair spreading. It is a nice styling aide and makes the hair slightly rigid. For weather changes Aloe Vera seals and protects the hair from winter damage. Aloe Vera contains all kinds of vitamins and proteins. PH restoration from aloe will help your hair with growth and moisture. Aloe reduces scalp fungus and other potential pathogens from invading the scalp. Add a little aloe for your pre-poo, and along with wheat germ and coconut milk creates a superb shine. Foot note 6

- Aloe Vera can act as a nice styling gel, and it may cause the hair to feel hard.

Kukui nut oil is oil similar to Noni and is found in Hawaii. Kukui oil is rich in Omega 3 and is commonly mixed with Macadamia oil. It penetrates easily and has soothing properties to help with sunburn, but it contains high levels of essential fatty acids like Linoleic acid. The linoleic oil absorbs easily into the skin and promotes tissue healing. Try this oil, and you will notice significant changes in your skin and scalp. This oil is excellent for people who suffer from any scalp disorder.

Coconut oil is one of the most commonly used oils. It is readily available and inexpensive. Coconut oil is one of the few oils that changes its molecular structure and becomes solid when cold. It adds the most protection and seals your hair, therefore, prevents dryness during seasonal changes. Not only is it cheap, but also a little amount goes a long way. Spoilage is not a problem if it is stored in a dark, cool, dry place. Thirsty, dull hair loves coconut oil.

This oil may last for days. Most naturals refer to it as their hair care staple. Coconut works well for pre-poo- just apply a minute amount to scalp and the ends of your hair before a shampooing.

Be forewarned over usage of most oil may increase acne, especially coconut oil. The preparation phase of washing your hair or pre-poo came from an Ayurvedic secret shared by the Indian culture.

The people of Indian use oils like coconut oil and Alma oil as a pre-poo. Alma is a bitter or sour fruit, which contains Vitamin C, which promotes the healing process. Ritualistic and cultural practices forbid any cutting of the hair. Hot oil treatments enriched with coconut oil prevents moisturizing deficits. To prevent splitting and breakage try the hot oil.

African-American women who wear their hair natural increase their use of coconut oil to seal and protect the ends to reduce breakage. It also reduces damage from the harmful process of shampooing. Coconut oil emulsifies for days. This oil is thick, and it stays on the hair shaft longer than any other oils. Split ends are common for everyone, and coconut will help reduce splitting.

- Coconut oil contains Vitamin E, Lauric acid, and it is one of the few oils that penetrate the shaft.

Lavender oil is used for calming and relaxation traditionally. This oil is an essential oil and should be mixed with a carrier oil to enhance the fullest benefits. Lavender also nourishes the hair, adds a small amount of moisturizer scalp and strands to help prevent shedding of the hair, improve circulation, and increase blood flow to assist in hair growth.

It also has an antiseptic property that reduces:

- o Fungus,
- o Bacteria,
- o Microbes,
- o Dry scalp.

Footnote 21

Burdock root oil is great for scalp relief. Dandruff is a common problem, and the use of Burdock root improves the quality of the scalp. Burdock root helps with Vitamin A and fatty acids production. It is a like maple or molasses, and it is not recommended for people with allergies, diabetes, and if you are pregnant. Footnote13

Burdock alone with birch, olive oil, horse tail, nettle, plantain oil has been documented to reverse thinning. Within 6-8 weeks you will notice an enormous amount of growth.   Burdock is high in Vitamin K, iron, and amino acids. People from Asia drink Burdock tea regularly.

Saw Palmetto - Through research for hair growth, it has been determined that permanent hair loss is created from certain hormone levels that trigger hair loss in the Anagen stage. Saw Palmetto can be found at the Vitamin local store or drug store. The plant is found commonly in California and the Atlantic coast. Saw Palmetto blocks the testosterone to DHT-Dihydrotestosterone, which cause's permanent alopecia.

MSM is another supplement that helps improve hair growth by increasing the Anagen phase. So, if you notice large areas where the hair is falling out. I recommend talking with your doctor or pharmacist to see if there are any interactions before adding this supplement to help reduce the hair loss. Some people noticed a significant difference in hair loss after the use of Saw Palmetto used topically. For oral use of the supplement, you should take Saw Palmetto at least 2-3 months before any significant difference will be noticed. And I must warn you that any vitamins supplement may potentially have effects on the liver, gallbladder, and the pancreas; so, make sure you are communicating with your healthcare providers regularly. Footnote 14

- Unlike Emu oil and Pumpkin oil, Saw Palmetto is one of the few oils that changes the DHT reproduction, and any use of it may increase your scalp appearance and reduce hair loss.

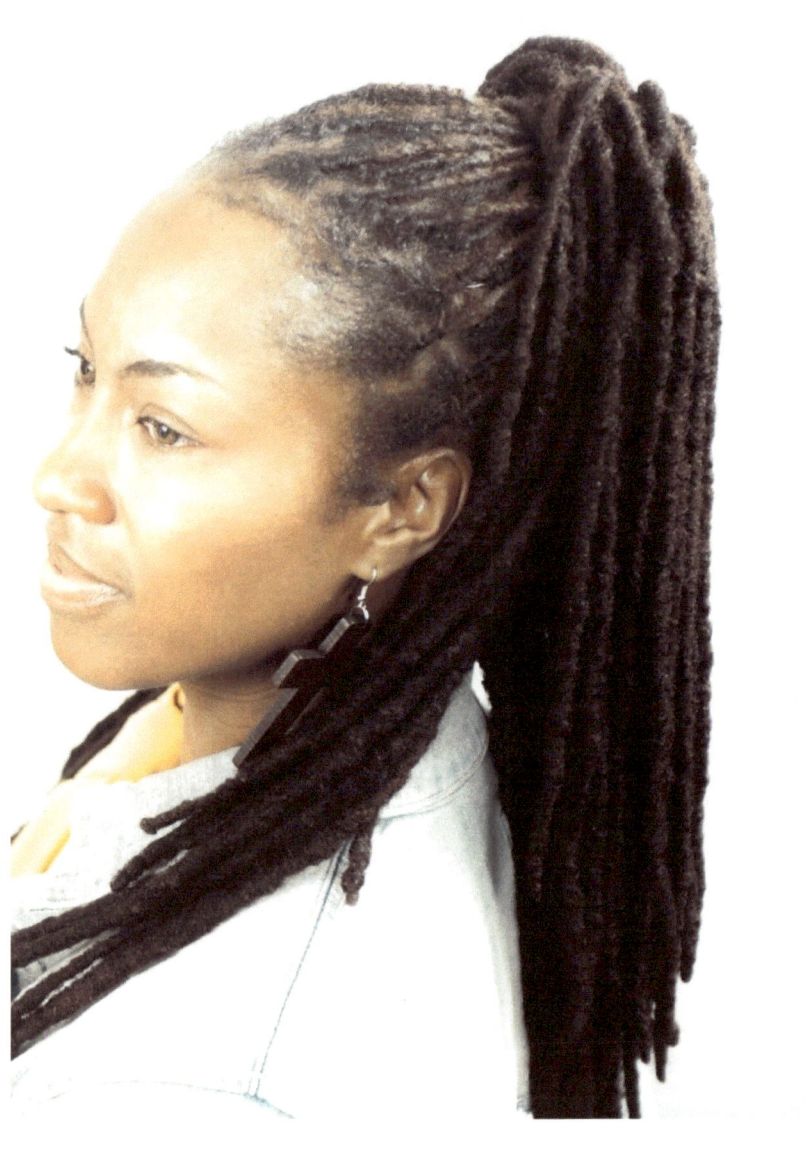

Stinging nettle has been around for centuries, and it works almost like Saw Palmetto in that it blocks the hormone production of DHT.

Also, DHT blocks our follicles from absorbing protein which causes the hair to become frail and shed.

Stinging nettle can be found in:

- Tea,
- Vitamins supplement,
- Oil.

Stinging Nettle is also known as Urtica Diocia. This is not one of the most pleasant fragrant oils, and I am not sure if you want to go around smelling like this oil. foot note 12

- Try the Stinging nettle oil in your scalp at night and cover the head with a bonnet and cleanse the scalp in the morning.

Castor oil is my all-time favorite oil because it is a humectant. People with low porous hair absorb moisture with most oils.

- Castor oil coats the hair nicely and lasts for about one week. After applying castor oil, no reapplication is necessary for 3-5 days.

- Castor oil is rich in Omega 6, Vitamin E, essential amino acids.
- It improves the hair growth.
- Castor oil reduces common problems of the scalp like dandruff caused by fungus and bacteria.
- The hair will appear very shiny after the use of castor oil.
- Castor oil is very inexpensive, and it can be used indefinitely without any potential effects on your organ or health. Footnote 11

Flax seed is an enriched Omega 3, fatty acid Alpha-Linolenic acid. Flaxseed is not only beneficial for your hair, but it reduces cardiac disease, Diabetes, and lowers your cholesterol. Flaxseed is well known for its antioxidant properties. This is one of the few oils that is a natural homeopathic great for the reduction in breast cancer and other cancers.

Cancer growths are driven by the production of estrogen. Off balanced hormone levels can cause so many health concerns like cancer, heart disease, stress, mental instability, and don't forget the aging process.

Flax seed oil - I love this oil because it can be converted from the seed form into a nice butter or gel. Flax seed oil is as beneficial as fish oil. Growth stimulation and healing properties for the inflamed scalp are why I explore flaxseed.

Flaxseed is rich with:

- B Vitamins,
- Magnesium,
- Potassium,
- Lection,
- Zinc,
- Protein,
- Omega 3
- Omega 6,

Studies have shown great benefits in the treatment of ADHD and arthritis. It helps lowers blood sugar and has great benefits on colon health. Try adding the seeds to your food, and you will notice a significant change in your bowel pattern. Flax seed lowers your risk of colon cancer.

- Try boiling flaxseed oil and draining it to create a nice gel.

Moroccan Oil

Moroccan oil and Argan oil reduce hair frizz. Argan oil is found and produced through a difficult process in Morocco. This oil is not produced in great volumes like other oils because of its limited trees source. It adds great luster, shine to the hair, and it great for hair growth also. It has some antioxidant properties and contains Vitamin E. It works a lot like the other oils in the prevention of scalp complication and dandruff. But both oils are very expensive and not produced in the United States. Be aware that most of these imported products contain preservatives, and you must pay a larger price to purchase 100% authentic Moroccan oil or Argan oil that may or may not be as potent by the time it reaches you in the United States.

- It has been said that anyone with 3c hair type (which is loose, softly coil hair) up to 4 hair type, (which is hard and has a tight coil to a coarse) may not get the best benefits from the use of either oil because the oil doesn't not always works for all hair types.

True Argan oil has little to no scent and must be stored in a cool dark place. I venture to say that by the time its gets to the US or your house, it may not be as beneficial as you think.

Footnote 10

Olive oil is easy, readily available oil that can be found almost anywhere. Olive oil works well for some people, but it is not growth-guaranteed oil. Although Olive oil is available everywhere, it is Mediterranean oil, and it has been used for centuries. This oil is high in fats. Olive oil repairs and invigorates the scalp by keeping it moisture. It works well in the prevention of split ends, and it is relatively inexpensive. Olive oil has antioxidant properties, and it is commonly used for sensitive hair. This oil is great for hair in so many ways because it is lightweight, and it is an emollient that contains Vitamin E.

- Olive oil is another fatty acid that works well to seal the follicles to improve the shine.

Grapeseed oil contains Linoleic, Oleic, and Stearic, Palmitic, Myristic, and Lauric.

- Myristic is a
  - Crystalline fatty acid,
  - Digestible
  - Non-toxic.

Oleic, commonly found in Emu oil, is a monounsaturated Omega-9 fatty acid. It can be found in animals and plants also.

Linoleic is an

- Omega 6,
- Vitamin E,
- Carboxylic acid,
- Essential fat.

Palmitic is a fatty acid found from animals and some plants.

Lauric acid is known to kill bacteria, virus, and fungus and it may be found in other oils like coconut oil. It is an essential fatty acid that is light, odorless, and used as a mild astringent. This oil cost is reasonable.

- Try Grapeseed oil if you are looking for a beautiful shine without the heavy weighted down effects of oil.

It is reasonable in cost. Grapeseed is great for strengthening your follicles.

Amla oil is commonly used in India. This oil strengthens the hair from the inside to the outer core of the hair. Generally, women prepare or pre-poo the hair the night before by applying the Amla oil to the entire head.

- This oil is not a pleasant in fragrance, but it adds great protein and moisture balance to the hair.

Upon awakening in the morning, you must shampoo the hair. Some African women have noticed no benefit to this treatment, and some have reported the combination of the Amla oil and their conditioner cause more shedding. So I would have to say you must be aware of combinations of different oils and protein that may alter the effect of what you are hoping to accomplish with the Amla oil.

Amla oil is ann essential fatty acid that binds with Iron and copper. It is not uncommon to see Fenugreek powder and Fenugreek oil mixed with Amla to improve the follicles and condition.

- It works ideal for the dry and itchy scalp.

Amla is generous with

- Vitamin C,
- Polyphenols,
- Flavonoid,
- Protein,
- Carbohydrates,
- Minerals,
- Antioxidants,
- Water.

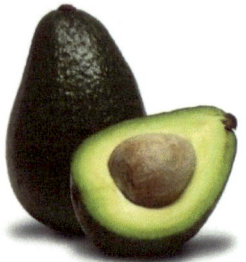

Avocado oil is a great oil for hair growth. It adds nutrients and vitamins to help you obtain a healthy scalp. I have a home hair care regimen I use to help me get the best benefit out of avocado oil. Try the avocado mask to help improve your hair growth today. This mask contains mashed avocado mixed with your favorite oil, honey, and yogurt.

This oil is a high monounsaturated fatty acid just like the olive oil and the jojoba oil.

It contains

- Lecithin
- Vitamin A,
- Vitamin D,
- Vitamin B6
- Amino Acids

- You will notice a remarkable difference in your hair when you use Avocado because it softens and creates more shine for your hair.

No matter what oil you use it is your choice, coconut and avocado oil works well for low porous 4 C hair, and this is my personal preference. There are several more oils that I did not discuss in this book, but I welcome you to share your favorite oils for more research.

Drink plenty of water

- Set a realistic goal of _____ (1000 cc) cups per days.
- Take hair Vitamins that include Biotin, Collagen, Vitamin B, Fe/ Iron.

Eat a healthy well-balanced meal.

- Add protein, fiber, vegetable, and fruits.

Exercise

- Set goal _5_ times per week.
- Try Yoga or the Inversion method- As mentioned in "Nubia's Guide to Going Natural."

Massage your scalp

- Try organic oil_____.

Shampoo and cleanse

- Pre-poo_____ times per week.
- Condition or co-wash_____ times a week.
- Clarify your hair twice a month- try Bentonite Clay, Black soap, or other natural cleansers.

Try less manipulating styles

- Change style every _____2-3 days.
- Avoid the heat, or try steam dryers instead.
- Avoid combing- finger detangle or use the Denman Brush.
- Detangle regularly while in the shower.

If hair growth is your goal, there are things you must know that may impede hair growth:

- Poor diet
- Poor handling
- Chemicals
- Traction Alopecia
- Inherited alopecia
- Areata Alopecia
- Split ends
- Too much tension
- Dryness
- Too much heat

Alternative treatment for alopecia:

- Stem cell
- Hair transplant
- Nonsurgical CRP
- Increase platelet rich plasma
- Rogaine
- You must see a dermatologist!!!!!!

For more information and guidance on natural hair care, please contact

Orjanette Bryant, author of Nubia's Guide to Going Natural

The Max Hydration Method

This method helps low porous, dry, brittle hair become more conditioned, less brittle, and during this process, the curls become more elongated and less shredding is noted. I like this method because my hair does not absorb protein, products, or conditioners during the shingling process, which is when you saturate each strand from root to tip with the product to stretch or elongate your curl pattern. The Max hydration method is a long, complicated process, and is recommended over seven days. I am unsure if there are any short cuts because I tried to use conditioners that were silicone based, products that are not plant base, and I never did the Cherry Lola protein treatment. But I want to expand the max hydration method to you so that can determine if this method is worth your time and investment. I will say Bentonite use and avoiding all shampoos have great results in my curls, and I am using much less oil.

Lisa Irby and Pinke Cube or Ms. DEEKAY, the known inspiration behind the Max Hydration Method.

Bentonite Clay for Detoxing

There are so many homeopathic ways to manage your hair care needs. Bentonite clay is by far one of my favorites. Bentonite is not dirt; it is clay from the volcanos enriched with calcium, potassium, sodium, and aluminum. Although most people think it must be export outside of the United States, in places like Mexico, it is also found in the Montana, and Wyoming or anywhere where there are volcano ashes. Another name for bentonite clay is montmorillonite clay. It improves eczema, dandruff, and other skin problems.

I use it to clarified, detox, and enhance the shine in my hair. There are so many variations on how to use the clay, but to simplify the process mix it with olive oil and water and add it to my favorite conditioners. It removes toxins, minerals, bacteria, and metals from my hair and leaves my hair elongated, soft and more manageable.

Make sure to select clay that is high quality to avoid the risk of clogging your pipes in the bathroom. Mixing the clay with vinegar works well to help improve skin.

1. They recommend 1:1 part one cup clay, water or (coconut water, rose water, or the Aloe Vera or liquid),

2. Only add one tablespoon of the ACV or the baking soda, and

3. Don't forget to add two tablespoons your oil of choice (olive oil, coconut oil, etc.)

Mixing the clay with baking soda also works great to help restore your ph. balance. The high-grade clay can be used to brush your teeth, skin care, and detoxification internally.

Great use for:

- Dogs with digestive problems

- Oral care- help remove the fluoride and toxins in your mouth.

- Skin care- help with skin disorders, acne, and eczema, skin, and staph infections

- Hair care- improves the skin and removes dandruff.

- Odor, bacteria, and parasites infections

- Colon health- only the liquid formula was recommended BECAUSE it works great to help detox your body.

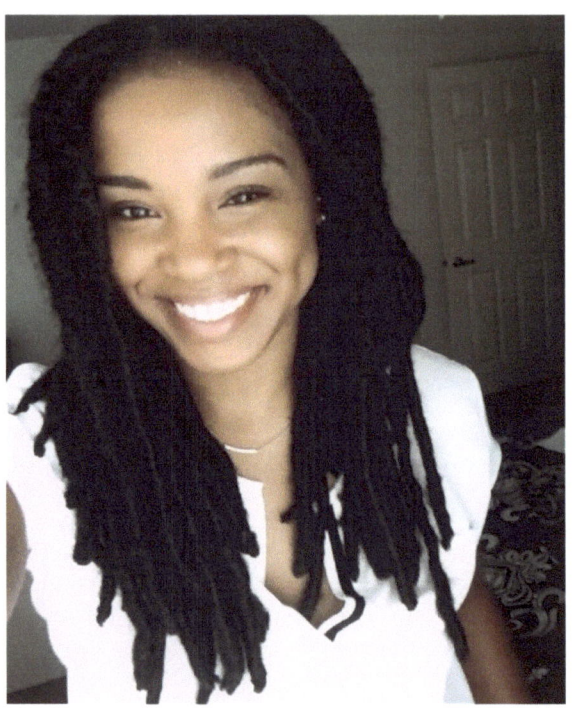

FAUX LOCS

Reference Sources

www.Altmedicine. about.com; footnote 1
www.stylecraze.com/?s=Vitamin+c; Source
www.Stylecraze.com/articles/amazing-benefits -of-vitamin-c-for-skin-hair-and-health/*; Footnote 2* www.Umm.edu/health/medical/
altmed/herb/burdock*;* Footnote 3 -
www.blackgirllonghair.com/2013/02/how-to-use-olive-oil-on-natural-hair/; Footnote 6
www.Naturallycurly.com/curlereading/kinky-hair-type-4a/5-ways-to-use-aloe-vera-gel/; www.longlocks.com*;*
http://site.thegreenlifeonline.org/2012/04/30/finding-a-safe-shampoo-and-what-ingredients-to-avoid/; Foot note 11- www. Med-health.net/Castor-Oil-For-Hair.html*;* Foot note 13-
www.Livestrong.com/sscat/vitamins-supplements/;
www.Nenonatural.com; www.Source voice.yahoo.com; Footnote 8- www.Supergrowlasers.com/vitamins-to-help-growth.php;Foot note 5 -www.Peppermintoilforhair.com; Foot note 28-
www.wheatgermbenefits.com/wheat-germ-oil/*;* Footnote 9 www.truehairgrowth.com; Footnote 15-
www.Judymcfarland.com/skin.shtml; Foot note 18-
www.Blackgirllonghair by cipriana Nov 28, 2011; Foot note 16-
Mayo Clinic and the www.Naturalstand.com to read more benefits of flaxseed go to mother Nature, University of Mary, and Medical Center March 14, 2009 (Steve Ehrlich), Harvard School of Public health, Herbal Power.; Foot note 20
www.Livestrong.com/sscat/vitamins-supplements/ *;*Footnote14 -
www.Sawpalmettohairlossreviews.com*;* Footnote 9-
www.truehairgrowth.com;   Footnote 12-
www.livestrong.com/article/138885-how-to-use-stinging-nettle-hair-loss/#page=1*;* http://www.iheartmyhair.com/back-basics-must-

styling-tools-curls-coils-kinks/; Footnote 6 - www.Naturallycurly.com/curleading/kinky-hair-type-4a/5-ways-to-use-aloe-vera-gel/; Footnote 20- www.livestrong.com/article/138885-how-to-use-stinging-nettle-hair-loss/#page=1; Footnote 11- www.Med-health.net/Castor-Oil-For-Hair.html; Foot note 17- www.Morocanoilreview.net; Footnote 8- www.Supergrowlaser.com; Footnote 25- www.livestrong.com/article/444501-does-vitamin-a-cause-hair-loss/#page=6; Footnote 27- www.Blackgirllonghair by cipriana Nov 28, 2011; Footnote 7- www.Peppermintoilforhair.com; www.Nenonatural.com; Foot note 21 www.urbanbushbabes.com; *Footnote 3-*www.blackgirllonghair.com/2013/02/how-to-use-olive-on-natural-hair/ *;* Footnote 29 www.Oilsofaloha.com/Kukui-skin-and Hair Care/; www.enslow.com; Footnote 29 www.mountainroseherbs.com/products/Kukui-nut-oil/profile ; www.Merriam-webster.com; www.supplementnews.org/ EPA; www.Umm.edu ; www.aoa.org; www.Natural news.com; www.dhs.wisonsin.gov; www.maxhydrationmethod.com; http://www.msdeekay.com/the-maxium-hydration-method-regimen http://www.historychannel.com.au/classroom/day-in-history/863/first-permanent-wave-%20for-hair-is-demonstrated http://www.ric.edu/faculty/rpotter/morgan.html http://www.revalid.com/all_about_hair/etymology.html http://durablehealth.net/bentonite-clay/bentonite-clay-for-hair-natural-hair-loss-benefits/ http://www.lipink.com/Health-Risks-in-Using-Your-Shampoo-s/5937.htm

All website resource sites are subject to the time they are researched

Book Sources

Super Natural Home by Beth Greer (Podale 2009)

Hair Care Millionaire by Edwin Brit Wyckoff (Enslow2011)

Madame CJ Walker, by Patricia Fredrick McKissack

The Hundred –Year- How to Protect Yourself from the Chemicals That Are Destroying Your Health by Randall Fitzgerald (A Plume Book 2006)

The Illustrated Herb Encyclopedia: A Complete Culinary, Cosmetic, Medicinal, And Ornamental Guide to Herbs, by Kathi Keville (Mallard Press 1991). Pp 33

The Way of Ayurvedic Herbs, by Karta Purkh, Singh Khalasa, and Michael Tierra (Lotus Press, 2008, pp 89, 162

The Illustrated Guide to Professional Hair Care and Hairstyles by Nicky Pope (South Water 2012) pp 10 -11

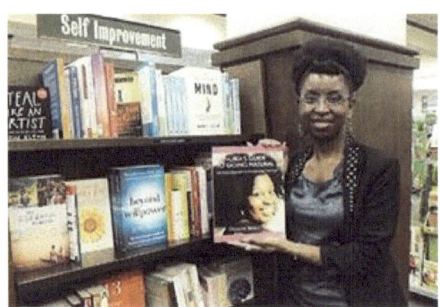

Author Orjanette Bryant obtained her degree in Science from Bethune-Cookman College.

She is a three-time published author and recently released *Small Voices Heard- The Parental Guide* with her son Dana Cooper.

Orjanette is a motivational speaker, wellness consultant, coach, business consultant, ministry, and a Registered Nurse. As a guest speaker on the panel at several Natural hair care events, she educates women about a chemical free approach to beauty. Through research and her interest in science, she shares her knowledge about natural hair care in her first publication book, *"Nubia's Guide to Going Natural."* You will learn the importance of avoiding the harmful chemicals and consider alternatives for your hair care.

Orjanette is an entrepreneur, and she supports her community through education and volunteering at several organization. As a director board member, she heads of the healthcare committee for the NAACP of Flagler County, Woman's advisory board for Bethune-Cookman College, Executive Committee for boy's foster home in Palm Coast, and director of Accel leadership training institute. Bryant explains her mentor, and biggest influence is her husband, Ron Bryant, a 25-year self-syndicated cartoonist, and animator.